FULL OF WATER

All the information you need regarding water and its effects on the body

FLEGRA

Table of contents

INTRODUCTION

Water is a material that exists in three different states: gaseous, liquid, and solid. It is made up of the chemical components hydrogen and oxygen. It is among the most abundant and vital substances. At room temperature, it is an odorless and tasteless liquid with a significant capacity to dissolve a wide range of other compounds. Water's flexibility as a solvent is, in fact, vital to all living things. Oceanic watery fluids are thought to have given rise to life, and living things rely on aqueous solutions for biological functions like blood and digestive juices.

There is water on other planets and moons in our solar system, as well as outside of it. Water seems colorless in small amounts, but it really possesses an inherent blue color due to a small amount of light that is absorbed at red wavelengths. Although it is a typical sight to see ice floating over water, this phenomenon highlights the peculiar chemical behavior of water, which is less dense when solid than when liquid. Despite having a simple structure, water molecules (H_2O) have very complex physical and chemical characteristics that set them apart from the majority of other substances on Earth. For instance, although it's normal to see ice cubes floating in a glass of cold water, chemical entities don't often behave in this way. Since the solid state of practically all chemical compounds is denser than the liquid state, the solid would sink to the bottom of the liquid. Since the ice that develops on ponds and lakes in cold climates serves as an insulating barrier to protect the aquatic life below, the fact that ice floats on water is very significant to the natural world. If ice were denser than liquid water, more water would be exposed to the cold when ice formed on a pond. As a result, all of the living organisms in the pond would ultimately perish from the freezing of the water.

Water moves between the ocean, the atmosphere, and the land surface throughout the hydrologic cycle. Relative water flows are shown by the numbers on the arrows. Under normal circumstances, water exists on

Earth's surface as a liquid, which makes it essential for enjoyment, transportation, and the support of a wide variety of plants and animals. Water may travel from the seas to inland regions via the atmosphere because it can easily transform into a vapor (gas), which condenses and feeds plant and animal life when it rains. Water has always had significant religious and philosophical significance in human history due to its prevalence.

Water is the only basic building block of matter, according to Thales of Miletus, who is sometimes credited with starting Greek philosophy in the sixth century BCE. Water is what makes up the earth, atmosphere, sky, mountains, gods, humans, beasts, birds, grass, trees, and even worms, flies, and ants, among other things. These are all distinct types of water. Ponder over water! Two centuries later, Aristotle still believed that earth, air, and fire were the other three basic elements and that water was one of them. For almost 2,000 years, people believed that water was a basic component. However, during the second half of the 18th century, investigations revealed that water is really a combination consisting of the elements hydrogen and oxygen.

Hoover Dam

The Hoover Dam, located on the Colorado River on the boundary between Nevada and Arizona, serves as an example of how water resources may be used for a range of uses, such as industry, agriculture, and human consumption. The majority of the water on Earth's surface (97.25 percent) is located in its seas, with the remaining 2.05 percent found in freshwater lakes, rivers, and groundwater. The remaining water is found in polar ice caps and glaciers. The importance of water recycling and purification rises with Earth's population and the need for fresh water. It's interesting to note that industrial water needs are often higher than residential standards for purity. For instance, high-pressure boilers need at least 99.999998 percent clean water. For the majority of applications, including human consumption, saltwater has to be desalinated due to the high concentration of dissolved salts it contains. This article discusses the physical, chemical, and molecular characteristics of water.

CHAPTER ONE

Water's structural makeup
Two hydrogen atoms and one oxygen atom make up a water molecule. Six electrons make up the outer shell of an individual oxygen atom, which has the capacity to store eight electrons in total. The outer electron shell of oxygen is filled when two hydrogen atoms are joined to an oxygen atom. Two hydrogen atoms joined to an oxygen atom by a single chemical bond make up the water molecule. The nucleus of the majority of

hydrogen atoms is made up entirely of protons. Water contains trace amounts of two isotopes: deuterium and tritium, whose atomic nuclei furthermore possess one or two neutrons, respectively. In addition to being used as a neutron moderator in some nuclear reactors, deuterium oxide (D_2O), often known as heavy water, is significant in chemical research. Despite having a seemingly simple composition (H_2O), water has very complex chemical and physical characteristics. Its melting temperature of 0 °C (32 °F) and boiling point of 100 °C (212 °F), for instance, are much greater than those of comparable compounds, such ammonia and hydrogen sulfide. Another peculiar characteristic of water is that it is less dense when it is solid, or ice, than when it is liquid. The electrical structure of the water molecule is the source of these aberrations. The water molecule has a unique bend instead of being linear.

structure of the water molecule showing the two hydrogen atoms bonded to the oxygen atom at an angle of 104.5 degrees of separation. The bond length, or O-H distance, is 95.7 picometers, or 3.77 × 10−9 inches (9.57 × 10−11 meters). The O−H bonds in the water molecule are polar, with the oxygen having a partial negative charge ($\delta-$) and the hydrogens having a partial positive charge ($\delta+$), due to the fact that an oxygen atom has more electronegativity than a hydrogen atom.

Droplets of water

Due to its polarity, water is drawn to other polar molecules. Water molecules stick together rather than to the surface, causing droplets, or beads, of water to form on a nonpolar surface. Water molecules include hydrogen atoms that are drawn to areas with a high electron density and have the ability to create weak connections, or hydrogen bonds, with those areas. This indicates that the nonbonding electron pairs of the oxygen atom on one neighboring water molecule attract the hydrogen atoms in that water molecule. It is thought that aggregates of water molecules constantly form and re-form to make up the structure of liquid water. The high viscosity and surface tension of water, along with other peculiar characteristics, are explained by this so-called short-range order.

Dividing water

water-dividing catalyst that releases oxygen and hydrogen. The outer (valence) shell of an oxygen atom has six electrons, with a maximum of eight electrons possible. An oxygen atom exchanges one electron of its own with the nucleus of another atom and gains a portion of that atom's electron when the two atoms establish a single chemical bond. The outer electron shell of the oxygen atom is filled when it forms a link with two hydrogen atoms. Ice structures Each oxygen atom in the solid state (ice) is surrounded by four hydrogen atoms, two of which are covalently bonded to the oxygen atom and the other two (at longer distances) are hydrogen bonded to the oxygen atom's unshared electron pairs. Intermolecular interactions produce this highly ordered but loose structure. Because of its open structure, ice has a lower density than liquid, where the ordered structure is somewhat disrupted and water molecules are generally closer together. Depending on the circumstances, a range of structures may form when water freezes. It is known that there are eighteen distinct types of ice that may be switched out simply altering the temperature and pressure outside.

Importance of liquid water's structure Water's liquid form has a very intricate structure that surely requires a great deal of molecular interaction. Larger values for characteristics like viscosity, surface tension, and boiling point are obtained from the substantial hydrogen bonding between the molecules in liquid water than would be predicted for a normal liquid with tiny molecules. For instance, water should boil at a temperature that is over 200 °C (360 °F) lower than what is actually seen because to the size of its molecules. Water molecules are highly correlated in their condensed forms (solid and liquid), yet they are comparatively independent at great distances from one another in their gaseous (vapour) phase. When aqueous solutions are formed, ionic substances dissolve mostly due to the polarity of the water molecule. Large volumes of dissolved salts are found in Earth's seas, and these salts are a valuable natural resource. Moreover, aqueous fluids are the site of hundreds of chemical processes that take place instantaneously to maintain the life of organisms. Furthermore, the solubility of ingredients like sugar and salt in water allows dishes to retain flavor during cooking. The interaction between the polar water molecules and the solute, or material being dissolved, is a significant factor in the solubility of compounds in water, despite the fact that it is a very complicated process. The positive ends of the water molecules are drawn to the anions when an ionic solid dissolves in it, whereas the negative ends are drawn to the cations. We refer to this process as hydration. A salt will usually dissolve in water due to the hydration of its ions. Strong water-ion interactions take the place of the strong forces that formerly existed between the solid's positive and negative ions throughout the dissolution process. Ionic materials separate into individual cations and anions upon dissolution in water. For example, the solution that forms when sodium chloride (NaCl) dissolves in water separates the Na+ and Cl– ions. A sodium ion's hydration Four molecules of water form a tight association with the sodium ion during the dissolution of sodium chloride. (Na+ has a hydration number of four.) A area where the presence of the hydrated ion [Na(H2O)4]+ partly orders the water molecules is located just outside this inner hydration sphere. This somewhat organized area mixes in with bulky, "regular" liquid water. In general, an ion's hydration number increases with its charge density—that is, its ratio of charge to surface area. Because of the increased crowding that happens when the hydrogen atoms of the water molecules are orientated toward the anion, negative ions often have lower hydration numbers than positive ions. In water, many nonionic substances also dissolve. For instance, the alcohol found in wine, beer, and distilled spirits, ethanol (C_2H_5OH), is very soluble in water. These drinks have different amounts of ethanol in an aqueous solution with additional ingredients. Because of the way the alcohol molecule is structured, alcohol is very soluble in water. The molecule can interact with water efficiently because it has a polar O-H bond, much like water. Water is not a suitable solvent for a variety of compounds. For example, animal fat is insoluble in pure water due to the incompatibility of fat molecules with polar water molecules resulting from their nonpolar nature. Ionic and polar compounds dissolve in water generally. "Like dissolves like" is a helpful guideline for figuring out if two chemicals are likely to be miscible, or will mix to produce a solution. That is, both two polar and two nonpolar chemicals have a high probability of mixing to produce a solution. Qualities and actions High-pressure and temperature water When water is heated to high temperatures and pressures, its typical behavior as a polar solvent (dissolving medium) alters. The molecules seem to interact with nonpolar molecules significantly more often as the water temperature rises. For instance, water possesses dissolving characteristics that are quite comparable to those of acetone (CH_3COCH_3), a popular organic solvent, at 300 °C (572 °F) at high pressure. Beyond its critical temperature and pressure

(374 °C [705.2 °F], 218 atmospheres), water shows notably peculiar behavior. Water loses its ability to be distinguished between its liquid and gaseous phases at its critical temperature. Instead, it transforms into a supercritical fluid, the density of which may be changed from liquid to gas by adjusting its temperature and pressure. Ionic solutes are easily soluble in supercritical water at high enough densities, much as in "normal" water. However, this supercritical fluid may also easily dissolve nonpolar compounds, which is not possible in ordinary water. Toxic wastes may be burned using supercritical

water as a combustion medium since it dissolves nonpolar compounds. For instance, waste organic materials may be combined with oxygen in supercritical water that is thick enough to ignite a flame that burns "underwater." With the benefit that a supercritical-water reactor is a closed system and doesn't release any emissions into the atmosphere, oxidation in supercritical water may be utilized to eliminate a broad range of dangerous organic compounds.

Characteristics

Physical characteristics

Water has a number of significant physical characteristics. The majority of water's physical characteristics are very unusual, even though these characteristics are well-known due to water's ubiquitous existence. Water has extraordinarily high levels of viscosity, surface tension, heat of vaporization, and entropy of vaporization due to the numerous hydrogen bonding connections that it contains, despite the low molar mass of its component molecules. Since ice has an open structure that maximizes hydrogen bonding, solid water has a lower density than liquid water, which is quite rare for a common material.

Certain physical characteristics of water

1.molar mass_ 18.0151 grams per mole

2. Melting point _ 0.00 °C

3.The boiling point: 100.00 °C

4.Maximum density (at 3.98 °C)&1,000,000 grams per cubic centimeter

5.Centimeter density (at 25 °C)_0.99701 grams per cubic centimeter

6. Vapor pressure (at 25 °C) _23.75 torr

7.Heat of fusion (0 °C) _ 6.010 kilojoules per mole 8.

8.Vaporization temperature (100 °C) _ 40.65 kJ/mol

9.The formation heat (25 °C) is equal to 285.85 kilojoules per mole.

10.Vaporization entropy (at 25 °C) _ 118.8 joules per °C mole

11.viscosity _0.8903 centipoise

12.Surface tension (at 25 °C) _71.97 dynes per centimeter

Chemical characteristics
Base-acid reactions

Numerous chemical reactions occur in water. The capacity of water to function as both an acid (a proton donor) and a base (a proton acceptor), which is a hallmark of amphoteric substances, is one of its most significant chemical characteristics. The best example of this behavior is when water is autoionized:

$$H_2O(l) + H_2O(l) \rightleftharpoons H_3O^+(aq) + OH^-(aq)$$

where (l) denotes the liquid state, (aq) denotes that the species are dissolved in water, and the two arrows show that the reaction can proceed in either direction and that an equilibrium condition exists. The concentration of hydrated H^+, also called H_3O^+ or the hydronium ion, in water at 25 °C (77 °F) is 1.0×10^{-7} M, where

M stands for moles per litre. As an equal number of OH– and H3O+ ions are generated, the OH– concentration at 25 °C is likewise 1.0 × 10–7 M. The H3O+ and OH– concentrations in water at 25 °C must always be 1.0 × 10–14: [H+][OH–] = 1.0 × 10–14, where [H+] denotes the hydrated H+ ion concentration in moles per liter and [OH–] denotes the OH– ion concentration in moles per liter. Both the acid and the water add H+ ions to the solution when an acid (a material that may create H+ ions) is dissolved in water. This results in a state where the concentration of H+ is higher than 1.0 × 10–7 M. The [OH–] must be reduced to a value less than 1.0×10^{-7} as it is a requirement that $[H+][OH-] = 1.0 \times 10^{-14}$ at 25 °C always hold true. The process $H+ + OH- \rightarrow H2O$ is the mechanism responsible for lowering the concentration of OH−. This reaction takes place to the amount required to bring the product of $[H+]$ and $[OH-]$ back to 1.0×10^{-14} M. As a consequence, $[H+] > [OH-]$, or more H+ than OH−, is present in the solution formed when an acid is introduced to water. When $[H+] > [OH-]$, a solution is considered acidic. The most often used technique to determine a solution's acidity is to measure its pH, which is expressed in terms of the concentration of hydrogen ions: pH is equal to -log [H+], where log represents the base-10 logarithm. The pH is 7.0 in pure water, where [H+] = 1.0 × 10–7 M. A solution with an acidic pH is one that is less than 7. When a base, or material that accepts protons, dissolves in water, the concentration of H+ decreases to the point where [OH–] > [H+]. The pH of a basic solution is greater than 7. To sum up, at 25 °C in aqueous solutions: impartial resolution [OH–] = [H+] pH = 7; [H+] > [OH–] in an acidic solution Baseline solution with pH

< 7 and [OH−] > [H+] pH greater than 7.

Reactions of oxidation and reduction

Flaming hydrogen gas is released when an active metal, like sodium, comes into contact with liquid water. This reaction is intense and produces heat. Using 2Na(s) and 2H2O(l), we get 2Na+(aq) + 2OH−(aq) + H2(g). An oxidation-reduction process, in which electrons are moved from one atom to another, is exemplified by this one. In this instance, water molecules get electrons from sodium atoms (creating Na+ ions) to create hydrogen gas and OH– ions. Similar interactions occur between the other alkali metals and water. Water reacts more slowly with less reactive metals. For instance, iron forms iron oxide and hydrogen gas significantly more quickly when it combines with superheated steam than it does with liquid water. Water: the chemical formula for iron states that it interacts very slowly with liquid water but very quickly with superheated steam to produce iron oxide and hydrogen gas. Noble metals, like silver and gold, have no reaction at all with water.

CHAPTER TWO

Benefits of water

We are kept lovely, content, and healthy by water. In addition to being one of the primary sources of life, it has several advantages, such as great skin and a faster metabolism. Additionally, it doesn't hurt to drink from an attractive bottle like the BKR bottle.

Here are fifty reasons to begin drinking right now.

1.Prevents the loss of fluids. Hydration is comparable to water;

therefore, this one should go without saying.

2.Eliminates poisons. Water is the most effective way to eliminate pollutants; forget about juicing. To enhance its advantages, add a slice of lemon to amp it up.

3.It makes the skin clear. Even though moisturizing is crucial, being hydrated from the inside out produces radiant skin.

4.Revives lackluster skin. You'll seem more alert and have brighter skin.

5.Prevents lip chapping. Water has more power than any lip balm, so bid adieu to dry lips.

6.Combats ashness. There are more options for treating ashy legs than just slathering on body lotion.

7.Reduction of weight. Of course, it has no calories!

8.It boosts the metabolism. For an increase in metabolism, start your mornings with a glass of cold water.

9.Facilitates digestion. Let constipation go.

10.It lowers the chance of illness. It essentially keeps your vital organs safe; therefore, we think that makes it extremely significant.

11.Provides headache relief. A migraine is never enjoyable. Drink some water since dehydration is often the cause of it.

12.Avoids cramping. Drink plenty of water—it really helps with your menstruation.

13.Maintains proper body temperature. Yes, the temperature of your body is determined by water. We perspire as a result!

14.Increases immunity. Drinking water is the most fundamental method to stay healthy, and nobody loves to become ill.

15.Boosts vitality. Get your legs moving, your arms pumping, your eyes blinking, and your fingers typing. You understand.

16.Optimizes exercise. Become your exercise partner's water if you haven't already.

17.Maintains fluid balance. Those bodily fluids are yin and yang.

18.Keeps cholesterol from rising. Just one more advantage of drinking water!

19.Electrolytes are restored. Drink some water instead of the sugar.

20.controls renal function. Give them some attention and stay hydrated; they depend on water to help filter the waste products in your body.

21.Keeps kidney stones at bay. Dehydration is the leading cause of kidney stones. Thus, sip away.

22.Lessens symptoms of a hangover. We like a good GNO, but not as much as the ensuing hangover. Alcohol causes your body to get dehydrated, so stay hydrated.

23.Enhances mental performance. It will stimulate your creative process.

24.Lifts the spirits. Everyone wants to feel happy, right?

25.Increases attentiveness. If just consuming water can enhance our senses, then we're all in.

26.Combats hypertension. Heart disease, blood clots, and strokes are just a few of the consequences of high blood pressure.

27.preserves joints. To drink water, not even the tiniest amount of elbow grease is needed.

28.It helps avoid hemorrhoids. Whoa, that's never enjoyable.

29.reduces traffic jams. Drink some H2O the next time your voice sounds nasal.

30.Lowers the chance of acid reflux. If you've never had the experience, count yourself fortunate.

31.Strengthens the heart. Joyful heart, joyful life!

32.Preserves pH equilibrium. To avoid sickness, our pH levels should be between 7.35 and 7.45. Drinking water helps to maintain a pleasant and healthy pH level.

33.Keeps osteoporosis at bay. In essence, this is the point at which your bones become brittle and delicate, making them more likely to shatter. Hurt.

34.Aids breathing. Drink plenty of water since breathing causes your body to lose natural water.

35.Enhances physical abilities. Whether you like jogging, yoga, or cycling, water will ensure that you get the most out of your exercise.

36.Handles back pain. Water consumption on a regular basis cushions your joints!

37.Prevents arthritis rheumatic. If our joints weren't working correctly, none of us would be moving like penguins.

38.treats urinary tract infections. You can tell whether you've been drinking enough water by the color of your urine!

39.Lowers ulcer risk. Ulcers are a different story altogether, even for those with a high pain threshold.

40.Enhances cognitive function. If you take good care of your brain, you'll be amazed at what it can do.

41.Assists with weariness. Yes, it does sound rather nice.

42.Distributes nutrients evenly throughout the body. Eating a clean diet is useless if you're not using the nutrients to their fullest.

43.Has an appetite-suppressive effect. Getting closer to our summertime figure? We're in!

44.Lessen asthmatic symptoms. You may not give much thought to the process of breathing, yet water is responsible for it.

45.Avoids wrinkles too soon. One thing is certain, however,water is maybe the most accessible miraculous anti-aging remedy available.

46.Controls salivary gland levels. It's important for your saliva to be able to complete its function of breaking down your meals.

47.Stops dental caries. Nobody enjoys going to the dentist. Beats foul breath

48.Even the strongest mint cannot compete with drinking water all day long.

49.Reduces edema. It's likely that you didn't drink enough water the night before if you discover that you wake up with swollen eyes or a swollen face.

50.Promotes relaxation. Anyone up for some water and chills?

The recommended daily intake of water for men and women is 15.5 cups (3.7 liters) for men and 11.5 cups (2.7 liters) for women, according to experts. However, your demands for water may change depending on environmental factors like temperature and other health issues. About 60% of your body is made of water. The body loses water continuously during the day, mostly via perspiration and urine, but it also loses water from breathing and other normal bodily activities. You need to consume a lot of water by eating and drinking every day to avoid being dehydrated. On the recommended daily intake of water, experts are divided. Previously, medical professionals advised eight 8-ounce glasses, or around 2 liters, or half a gallon, every day. The 8×8 rule refers to this and is quite simple to recall.

However, several medical professionals now advise drinking water continuously throughout the day, even if you're not thirsty.

Like most things, each person's experience will vary. In the end, a variety of internal and external variables determine how much water you need.

How much water is necessary?

The amount of water required varies from person to person and relies on several factors. The U.S. National Academies of Sciences, Engineering, and Medicine's general advice for adults is focused on:

For women, 11.5 cups (2.7 liters) each day

For males, 15.5 cups (3.7 liters) every day

This includes liquids from meals, drinks, and juices, as well as from water. The items you consume provide you with 20% of your total water intake on average.

It's possible that you need more water than others. The amount of water you need also varies.

•Where you are residing: In hot, muggy, or arid climates, you will need extra water. If you live in the mountains or at a high altitude, you'll also need extra water.

•Your diet: You may lose more water via increased urine if you consume a lot of coffee and other caffeinated drinks. If a large portion of your diet consists of spicy, salty, or sweet meals, you may also need to drink extra water. Alternatively, if you don't consume many items high in water content, such as cooked or fresh fruits and vegetables, you should drink extra water.

•The season or temperature: Because you perspire more in hot months than in colder ones, you could need more water.

•Your surroundings: You may get thirsty more quickly if you spend more time in the sun, in warm weather, or heated indoor spaces.

•How active you are: Compared to someone who sits at a desk all day, you will need more water if you move, stand, or are otherwise physically active throughout the day. You will need additional fluids to replace lost water if you exercise or engage in any other strenuous activity.

•Your health: You should drink extra water if you have a fever or illness, or if you lose fluids due to diarrhea or vomiting. You will also need extra water if you have a medical condition like diabetes.

Diuretics are one kind of drug that may cause water loss.

•Being pregnant or nursing: To keep hydrated, you should drink more water if you are expecting or nursing a child. After all, your body is working for two or more people.
The amount of water you need to keep healthy depends on several variables, including your surroundings, activity level, and health.

-Is there a relationship between water consumption and brain activity?

Many individuals assert that dehydration throughout the day causes a decline in both energy levels and cognitive function.

Earlier research conducted on females revealed that a 1.36 percent fluid loss after exercise decreased mood and attention and increased headache frequency.

A more recent research conducted in China with 12 male university students discovered that going 36 hours without drinking water had a discernible impact on short-term memory, weariness, concentration and focus, and response time.

Physical performance may be impacted by even minor dehydration. When your body loses more water than it takes in, it becomes dehydrated, which may lead to symptoms like headaches and exhaustion. A 1 percent loss of body water was shown to hurt the strength, power, and endurance of the muscles in clinical research including older, healthy males.
Even while 1% of body weight loss may not seem like much, it represents a considerable loss of water. This often occurs when you don't drink enough water,

perspire a lot, or are in a heated environment.

Your physical and mental well-being may suffer from mild dehydration brought on by physical activity or hot weather.

-Does consuming a lot of water aid in weight loss?
Many people suggest that increasing your water intake will help you lose weight by speeding up your metabolism and decreasing your hunger.
Studies have shown that higher-than-average water consumption is associated with

lower body weight and body composition scores.

Chronic dehydration was linked to obesity, diabetes, cancer, and cardiovascular disease, according to another analysis of research.

In previous research, scientists calculated that consuming 68 ounces (2 liters) of alcohol in a single day led to a thermogenic response, or a quicker metabolism, which raised daily energy expenditure by around 23 calories. Although little at first, the sum has the potential to grow . You may cut down on calories by sipping water around 30 minutes before to eating. This may occur because the body may easily confuse thirst for hunger.

People who drank 17 ounces (500 mL) of water before each meal lost 44% more weight over 12 weeks than those who didn't, according to a 2010 research conducted on middle-aged and older individuals. More recently, research on young men revealed that those who drank around 19 ounces (568 mL) of water before each meal were required to eat less during the meal to feel full.

All things considered, it seems that consuming enough water, especially before meals, may help you better control your hunger and maintain a healthy body weight, especially when paired with a balanced diet.

Furthermore, there are several additional health advantages of drinking plenty of water.
Water consumption will temporarily raise your metabolism somewhat, and it can help you cut down on calorie intake when you drink it 30 minutes before each meal.
For some individuals, weight reduction might be facilitated by both of these benefits.

-Is drinking more water a good way to stay healthy?

Your body needs to drink enough water to operate normally. Increased water consumption may also be beneficial for the following health issues:

- Constipation: Drinking more water helps alleviate constipation .

-Urinary tract infections: New research indicates that drinking more water may help shield the urinary system and bladder from recurrent infections.

-Kidney stones: Although more research is required, an earlier study found that a high hydration intake reduced the incidence of kidney stones.

-Skin hydration: Research indicates that drinking more water improves skin hydration, but further studies are required to determine if this also affects acne and improves clarity.

Constipation, kidney stones, bladder and urine infections, and skin dryness are just a few of the health issues that may be alleviated by increasing water consumption and maintaining proper hydration.

-Are other liquids included in your total?

There are other beverages than plain water that support your fluid balance. Other meals and drinks may also have a big impact.

One misconception is that since caffeine is a diuretic, it doesn't help you stay hydrated. This is true for tea and coffee, for example.

Research indicates that these drinks have little diuretic action, although some individuals may have increased urination as a result.

But even beverages with caffeine contribute to your body's total water intake.

In varied amounts, water may be found in most meals. Water may be found in meat, fish, eggs, and particularly in fruits and vegetables.

Water-rich meals and coffee or tea together may support the maintenance of your fluid balance. Other drinks, such as tea and coffee, may also help maintain fluid balance. Water is also present in most meals.

Signs of dehydration

You must preserve the water balance to survive.

Your body thus has a highly developed mechanism to regulate when and how much you drink. Thirst sets in when your body's overall water content drops below a certain threshold. You don't have to think about this; breathing-like systems take care of this for you.

Your body is capable of regulating its water balance and letting you know when to drink more.

Even while thirst is a good sign of dehydration, feeling thirsty alone may not be enough to support good health or performance during physical activity.

You could already be experiencing the negative symptoms of

dehydration, including headaches or weariness, when thirst hits.

It may be more beneficial to use the color of your pee as a gauge to determine how much you're drinking. Urine should be clean and pale.

The 8×8 rule is unscientific and has been refuted by prior studies. There may be situations when drinking more water is necessary.

The most significant one could occur when perspiration is heavier. This involves physical activity and hot temperatures, particularly in arid regions.

If you perspire a lot, you may replace the fluid you've lost with water. Long-term, high-intensity exercisers may also need to resupply water and electrolytes, such as sodium and other minerals.

During pregnancy and nursing, your body needs more water. Additionally, you need extra water when you have a fever, diarrhea, or vomiting. Increase your water consumption as well if you want to lose weight.

Additionally, as individuals age, their thirst processes may fail, so older adults may need to be particularly mindful of how much water they drink. Adults over 65 have an increased risk of dehydration, according to studies.

Since the body naturally detects thirst, most individuals don't need to pay too much attention to how much water they drink.

Nonetheless, there are situations when paying closer attention to how much water you're drinking is necessary.

-How much water, according to your age and weight, should you drink?

It's advised by experts to drink enough water to get a light yellow urine color. There is no hard-and-fast guideline for the precise quantity of water to drink since it may vary based on variables beyond these. You may need to drink more water than you would normally require in particular situations, such as when you perspire or have certain medical problems.

-Is drinking a gallon of water per day excessive?

For men, the recommended daily consumption of water is somewhat less than one gallon. It is a little over 4 cups less for women. Depending on several circumstances, including the temperature, your level of activity, and if you are pregnant or nursing, your specific water requirements may exceed the recommended amount.

In summary

Nobody can ultimately determine how much water you need. Numerous elements are involved in this.

To find out what works best for you, try experimenting. While some individuals find that drinking more water than normal improves their performance, others find that it only makes them need to use the restroom more often.

These rules should apply to most individuals if you wish to keep things simple:

Have enough fluids throughout the day to produce pale, clear urine.

Drink when you are thirsty.

Make careful efforts to stay hydrated, especially during periods of excessive heat, while exercising, and at other indicated times. That's it!

CHAPTER THREE

What Takes Place If You Consume Too Much Water? (Intoxication by Water);

The body Nevertheless, several medical experts now recommend drinking water constantly throughout the day, even if you don't feel thirsty.

Everybody will have a different experience, as with most things. The amount of water you need is ultimately determined by several internal and environmental factors.

We rely mostly on water to operate properly, yet consuming

too much of it too quickly might have detrimental effects on one's health. Only 0.8 to 1.0 liters of water can be eliminated by the kidneys in an hour, and an excessive water intake might throw off the body's electrolyte balance.

Accidentally consuming too much water is rare, although it does occur sometimes, generally as a consequence of dehydration after rigorous exercise or competition.

General signs of water intoxication include nausea, vomiting, confusion, and disorientation.

Rarely, water intoxication may result in cerebral edema and even death.

The symptoms, causes, and consequences of water intoxication are discussed in this article. It also examines the recommended daily intake of water for each individual.

Water Toxicity: What Is It?
There are several terms for water toxicity, including overhydration, hyponatremia, water intoxication, and poisoning.
One of the main problems associated with water toxicity is its effect on sodium levels, which are

essential electrolytes for your body. Sodium is essential for sustaining blood pressure and for the healthy operation of your muscles, neurons, and other bodily tissues, according to the U.S.

Water Toxicity: What Causes It?
Although consuming too much water is often the cause of water toxicity, the Cleveland Clinic notes that hyponatremia may also result from excessive salt loss from the body on a less frequent basis. These reasons may consist of:

•Using diuretics. You may excrete more sodium as a result of them.

excessive alcohol consumption. You may urinate more as a result of this and lose fluids due to vomiting.

•Experiencing untreated diarrhea. Dehydration and decreased sodium levels might result from this.

•Making use of certain drugs. Hyponatremia may be exacerbated by some medications, such as carbamazepine (Tegretol) and selective serotonin reuptake inhibitors (SSRIs).

In addition, individuals shouldn't be afraid to consume water for fear of being contaminated by it. Although this is a very uncommon occurrence, it's still a good idea to be prepared for it. Your thirst is a useful indicator, so follow it.

-What are Excesses in Water Consumption?

The quantity of water that is considered excessive depends on factors including age, height, weight, and degree of physical activity. According to the US National Academies of Sciences, Engineering, and Medicine, the recommended daily fluid consumption is 3.7 liters for males and 2.7 liters for women. However, according to the Mayo Clinic, food typically accounts for 20% of this. Depending on lifestyle choices, individual health, exercise habits, and the local environment, this quantity may be either little or too much for certain people.

Utilize calculations based on your weight and level of activity to ascertain the ideal water consumption for you. To calculate your daily fluid consumption in ounces, divide your body weight in pounds by two if you are not exercising. To convert this to milliliters, multiply the number by 29.6. If you exercise, use the same technique but be sure to include the water lost via activity by measuring your weight both before and after. You should consume 16–20 oz (0.5–0.6 liters) of water for every pound (0.45 kg) lost.

-What Happens If You Drink Too Much Water?

Drinking too much water may cause a variety of problems, from minor ones like frequent urination to moderate ones like cramping and vomiting to major ones like seizures that can be fatal in cases of acute, short-term water intoxication. However, the long-term consequences of persistent overhydration are not well-documented in medical literature.

Overhydration may be equally as hazardous as dehydration, although being relatively uncommon. For this reason, it's important to consume the recommended quantity of water each day to prevent any negative health effects.

-What Signs Of An Excessive Water Intake?

Your brain expands when you drink too much water too quickly because you dilute the electrolytes in your blood—especially the sodium—which promotes the flow of water into brain cells. Your brain may have a "major problem" as a result of this enlargement.

The Cleveland Clinic states that this may result in a wide range of possible symptoms, such as:
-Urine's color
-frequency of bathroom trips
-consuming water is not necessary
-vomiting
-Headaches
-Weary
-low glycemic level
-cramping in the muscles
lips, hands, and feet without color
-Feeling sleepy
-dual vision
-Perplexity
-breathing difficulties

-Convulsions

-Seizures, comas, and even death may result from severe water poisoning.

-Why Is Water Intoxication Associated With Electrolyte Loss?

Water intoxication and electrolyte loss are associated because too much water dilutes the body's natural reserves of salts, including electrolytes. If athletes feel they may have been dehydrated following physical exertion, they may replenish electrolytes with certain high-TDS mineral waters or sports beverages. According to a Cleveland Clinic Foundation journal article, these beverages won't assist if the water intoxication has become too bad.

A doctor's visit is not enough if you are suffering symptoms like altered mental state or seizures. You need to get help immediately.

DEHYDRATION (not drinking enough water).
Approximately two-thirds of the human body is composed of water. Water is an essential

element for life, since it aids in blood circulation, lubricates joints and eyes, and eliminates waste products and pollutants. Insufficient water intake has the potential to escalate into a medical emergency. Read this informative blog to learn about the causes of dehydration and how to avoid it.

-Dehydration: What Is It and Why Does It Happen?

When your body doesn't have the necessary quantity of fluids to operate correctly, dehydration sets in. Although the human body routinely loses and uses up water via perspiration, urination, bowel movements, salivation, and tears, an imbalance may result in the body if more fluids are lost than are replaced. Dehydration is more harmful when it affects little children and elderly people. It may vary from mild to moderate and potentially reach severe or catastrophic levels.

Aside from not drinking enough water, other frequent causes of dehydration are as follows:
-Sweating excessively
-more frequent urination than normal
-diarrhea
-vomiting
-High temperature
-Some drugs, including diuretics

-Chronic conditions such as diabetes, renal problems, and cystic fibrosis.

We sometimes forget to hydrate ourselves because we are too preoccupied with our everyday activities. Furthermore, we might lose awareness of the need for fluids for our bodies. In any case, there are several indicators you should watch out for to determine when you need to restock.

Mild to moderate dehydration symptoms include:
-Urine with a dark yellow color
-Mouth that is sticky or dry
-Desiccated skin

-Headache
-Not as much peeing as normal

Severe dehydration symptoms include:
-lightheadedness
-Dark yellow pee
-Extremely parched skin
-Losing consciousness
-Accelerated heart rate and
-Breathing
-Fatigue or drowsiness
-Sunken eyes

How to Stay Hydrated

Even while over-the-counter medications purchased at a pharmacy may help prevent and sometimes even cure dehydration, you should always seek medical assistance if you think you may be suffering from severe dehydration.

Among the strategies to stop dehydration from getting to the point of danger are:
- Making sure you are aware of any potential dehydration symptoms
-As soon as your body indicates that you are thirsty, pay attention to it.
- Examining the hue of your pee; a dark yellow tone indicates dehydration.
-Drink a glass of water as soon as you wake up, as it has been at rest

and you haven't had access to water.

-Eating foods high in water content, such as iceberg lettuce, cherries, celery, and melons

-Drinking more water while you're unwell, working in the heat, or exercising

-Including drinks with electrolytes as necessary (avoid drinks with a lot of sugar).

-Choosing other drinks over water if it's not easily accessible